MW00477126

SCARS

This small book contains a large story about the repercussions of combat, not only in the lives of our military men and women, but also in the lives of their loved ones, families and friends. It is a story about PTSD and mild concussions and how these combat scars affect relationships and spirituality.

SCARS

The Effects of Post Traumatic Stress on Family, Relationships and Work

Peace,

Richard Berg, csc

by Richard Berg, CSC

SCARS
The Effects of Post Traumatic Stress on
Family, Relationships and Work

Copyright@ 2013 by Richard F. Berg

All rights reserved. No part of this book may be used or repro-
duced in any manner whatsoever without the written permission
of the publisher.

10 9 8 7 6 5 4 3

ISBN 978-0-9859377-5-1

Published by
CORBY BOOKS
A Division of Corby Publishing, LP
P.O. Box 93
Notre Dame, In 46556
www.corbypublishing.com
(574) 784-3482

Distributed by
ACTA PUBLICATIONS
4848 N. Clark Street, Chicago, IL 60640
800-397-2282
www.actapublications.com

Manufactured in the United States of America

Foreword

The privilege of intimate conversations with courageous men and women who have served in combat opens minds and hearts to what they endure in war and the cross they bear upon their return home. Their openness with me leaves me feeling both inspired and in awe. I serve as a licensed professional counselor working with active and retired military service members who suffer from Post Traumatic Stress Disorder (PTSD) and chemical dependency issues. Most of these men and women are still on active duty and arrive at our treatment facility after going through a major crisis, usually related to their difficulty readjusting to life after returning home on leave or from deployment.

Father Richard Berg, CSC, asked me for permission to visit some of our service members as he wanted to learn more about the impact of PTSD upon relationships and spirituality. His request was granted as I could not think of a more understanding, empathic, and compassionate person to visit these men and women. After several interviews with soldiers, Richard Berg shared with me how deeply touched he was by the way these individuals shared their inner lives in remarkable ways and that these sessions always left him with hope and courage.

One day when I contacted Father about visiting a few more soldiers, he informed me that the idea of writing a story to help people understand PTSD came to him during these interviews. The characters in this story, he told me, would reflect the lives of many service members. As he began writing, he enlisted the support and ideas of nine of our soldiers to help him develop the characters and the story based on real life and actual events.

In reflecting on this story about SCARS from life and combat and the lives of men and women I work with, I continue to be overwhelmed by the devastation of war. Words can never fully describe the cross our military members and their families bear. However, I am humbled by the Christ within all of these men and women who are willing to give their lives for others.

Here, then, is the story of the soldiers I work with, and those Father Berg interviewed.

~ Ben Cobb, LPC

PART ONE

Deployment

CHAPTER 1

ERIC

Mom shouted, "Eric, get down here." I was nearly finished getting my stuff together. In a way, I told myself, I don't feel like being downstairs. "Eric?" She really didn't sound her usual self trying to disguise her stress. Tonight was not a night anyone was looking forward to. I heard our guests arriving. Noise from the kitchen signaled dinner was almost on the table. I got into my uniform and shoes, closed my eyes, and took a deep breath. This was my last night at home for a very long time. Thank goodness.

I wanted them to see me in my military uniform. I remember how my girlfriend Emilee, my best friend Jim and a few relatives awkwardly strained to think of what to say to me....After a year and where I have been, I don't have much recollection about what they said or tried to say that evening. I remember feeling their apprehension, watching their wary eyes, realizing how guarded these goodbyes were for them, and for me.

The fragrances of the roast turkey dinner and fresh-cut flowers filled our house. The scent reminded me of our Thanksgivings, but tonight was not a Thanksgiving. Mom put the finishing touches on the table set for nine and it gleamed with Grandmother's best china and silver. Mom's aunt, who is Sister Mary Agatha, was in the kitchen making the gravy. Emilee, shy and avoiding my eyes tonight, was forcing smiles and helping with the drinks. Truthfully, this was not the easy evening I hoped for. It seemed anything but that.

Conversations at dinner were muted. Aunt Agatha poured wine and served dinner. Emilee and Jim helped her in the kitchen. I noticed a few wet eyes as Mom was reassured by all of their love and help. Caring for our orchard and vineyard would be her burden now. They pledged their support. Back then I was hoping Jim could find a way to help her. He was out of school that year and could use a job.

When I was in the kitchen I overheard someone say, "Roberta, we are so proud of Eric." From the doorway I watched them force smiles and nod. This seemed to signal the gift-giving. I sat down and didn't say a word. They handed me a little package with an American flag pasted on it. Inside I found pictures of everyone at the table in a tiny album and a medal of St. Joseph I kept in my pocket in Afghanistan.

Our dinner celebration ended with a few toasts and hidden fears.

At 2:30 in the morning our staff sergeant from New-berg came to get me. Because of the stormy weather, we left early to be on time for formation at the armory in Woodburn.

CHAPTER 2

ROBERTA

The next morning I woke up with "pride" on my mind. Those words, "Roberta, we are proud of Eric," rang true, no doubt, but they were directed to me, not to Eric. Alarmed all those months that his Oregon National Guard unit was called up for medical support in Afghanistan, I didn't think much about being proud. Like every other mother, I worried. Truthfully, I was not always proud of Eric or myself. But I'll get to that later, after telling you about the morning after his departure.

I suspected the day would be like this as I opened the curtains. Our valley turned totally white. The sun rising over the hillside touched bare trees and they glistened. Nothing stirred. It did seem beautiful but felt very, very cold, frozen. We rarely have these severe snowstorms in western Oregon, perhaps only two or three in ten years. So everything comes to a standstill. I remember the morning was unwelcome, chilling and bitter. That's what I felt after Eric left, and that's what I'll never forget. Thinking back, I suppose I was ill prepared for this first day and for the months ahead. I told myself to face up to having him gone and to do my best. This was not going to be easy.

I put on my bathrobe and warmed a little. The smell of sizzling bacon and fresh coffee beckoned me downstairs. Agatha was fixing breakfast. Always serving others, she has been such a good friend over the years—more than just my aunt—always someone I could count on, a dependable mainstay of counsel and wisdom. We chatted. "Agatha, I worry for Eric. He's been through so much growing up, you know, especially the ordeal with his father." She listened intently and nodded knowingly.

When she was cleaning up after dinner last night, Agatha found a mysterious sealed envelope which she handed to me. "What's this?" I asked. I imagined Eric must have put this on the table before he left in the pre-dawn. It looked like his writing. It read, "Do not open this yet." I held the envelope up to the light and told Agatha, "I can't see what's in it. I'll have to ask him about this when he calls." I placed the envelope back between the salt and pepper.

Agatha listened to my worries about keeping the filbert orchard and vineyard going without Eric's help. "If we get a decent harvest of grapes and the trees do well again this year, I'll be able to make it. I hope so. But, Agatha, we need to get you a ride to Portland."

Jim answered the phone. "Yes, Roberta, I'll be glad to drive Sister Agatha to town. We'll be careful for you. I've driven in worse without any problem."

CHAPTER 3

JIM

Sister Agatha and I headed down the icy road. It took too long for the heater to warm the car. As it did, I mentioned how frozen everything outside must feel. "You know, Jim," Sister replied, "in the winter these bare trees are still filled with life, especially at their roots." I looked over and smiled. "I wish I could say the same for myself, Sister. You know, it'd be nice if I could find more life at the core of myself. I've been thinking about stuff…problems I haven't solved. Eric tried to help me some, but I still have questions. Do you think we can find answers in our roots?" Agatha laughed. "What an interesting thought! Let's see, my own roots extend to my family and friends—and to my work at the college—and to my spiritual life, too. I never gave much thought to having human roots like these with answers!"

I could tell she was a person I could talk to. "Now that I'm twenty-one I can take a job at the The Mustang, that bar in McMinnville. I've been there a few times. The owner told me he needs a bouncer and offered me the job." "A bouncer?" she asked. "Yes, the place gets pretty unruly, especially on weekends, and he needs help." "You don't look like the bouncer type to me, Jim. Are you sure that's your kind of work?" "I can fight, not just scrap, but really fight. You know Dad was the principal at our elementary school and whenever he punished guys, they took it out on me. I used to go home and cry! Then, I made up my mind to stand up for myself. So I took martial arts lessons and became a good fighter. So, the bullying at school stopped when I turned into a bully. I guess you could say I became what I hated most: a bully."

She must have thought that, since I'm so thin, I didn't have the strength to do the job. That's actually one of my strengths. People don't expect me to be the enforcer type. I explained: "But the extra strength I have is also a problem for me. It is anger." I told her about my short fuse and powerful explosions! She winced. "One night Eric and I were drinking at that bar. In fact, both of us were drunk. Eric looked over at me and smiled. I said, 'What the hell are you smiling about?' I hit him, knocked him onto the floor, and kicked him. You know if he hadn't been drunk, I think I could have really hurt him. It was terrible. I felt so guilty. You know, Eric's my best friend. So, now what do I do? I drink to calm my anger. Beer's my medicine. The only one I know."

There. I let her in on my troubles. Thank goodness she didn't have much to say, but I wanted us to talk about this again. I hoped so.

CHAPTER 4

AGATHA

I arrived home worn out. At luncheon the only conversation around our convent table was the weather and cancelled classes. Since no one seemed able to make it into work, I made my way—carefully—to my office in the library not too far away. Six phone messages waited for me; most of these telling me, "I'm sorry, Sister, I can't get to the College today; I'm snowed in." I could have opened the library that afternoon but decided otherwise. It is more compassionate to give people a reason not to risk it.

A lot of business had piled up on my desk, so I sat there catching up and also pondering how I could possibly continue to be of help to Roberta, Eric and Jim. I thought to myself, I can support them by listening, and certainly with my prayer. I wish I could do more. Maybe that will happen. I don't know. I think letting them tell me their stories could help. No doubt about it, I'll need to get Jim's trust if I'm going to be able to help him into AA. It might be good to send cards with simple messages or perhaps a good book about the way others solve problems. These would be small gestures and a good start.

I'm usually pretty good at falling asleep. But not tonight! My conversation with Jim this morning keeps crossing my mind over and over. I rehearse what he told me a few times. I imagine the fight he had with Eric and this brings a few tears to my eyes. If I wake up during the night, one of my habits is to pray for whoever comes to mind. Tonight my family and their friends flood my mind, especially Roberta and Eric, then Jim, then Emilee. First, I think a bit about each one, and then ask God to bless her or him, and send my own love their way through God. Sometimes, during the night, I might pray for twenty or thirty people whom God brings to my mind before I fall back to sleep. I find it's better than counting sheep!

When I wake up in the morning, I often have a new insight about something or someone. Now and then the questions I take into the night seem answered or solved. It's very special to know my mind and heart are at work during sleep. One of my going-to-bed prayers is, "Lord, continue to teach me through the night that I may know you better, love you more and do your work. Amen."

I am happy to report to you it works!

CHAPTER 5

EMILEE

Saying goodbye was really, really hard. I love Eric and I know he loves me. He told me he did at the bonfire. We've even talked about getting married when he gets back from Afghanistan. That's our dream. I'm getting to know his mother and friends better and, now that he's gone, I will spend more time with them. My own family broke up when I was four years old, and I am an only child raised by my grandparents. They are generous, good and wonderful people. They're still pretty backward when it comes to dating and, while I think I needed to be watched over when I was a girl, now I'm a woman and I know what I'm doing. Before Eric left I took him over to see them and they seemed pleased to meet him. They were happy/proud that he was being deployed. Service men are really respected by their generation. Anyway, I know I won't be dating until he gets back.

If I could get closer to Roberta by working for

her, she will grow to love me like Eric does. She's been through a lot, and I think she'll feel stranded being alone at home with all the work facing her. I could help with the vineyard and even find some people I know in town to work in the orchard. I'm more cut out for work outdoors and so, when spring comes, I can quit my job at the grocery and go to work for her. I think I'll have a serious talk with her soon.

When Eric talked about his dad, all he could say was, "When I was just a kid I was scared to death of him, especially when he was drinking. I can't count the times I had to escape from him. I'd run outside and climb up a tree as fast as I could, up where he couldn't reach me."

It's a shame that Eric was so mistreated by his father. No one mentions this, as far as I know, but he let me in on this secret. He keeps it very close to the vest. Most of the time, he tells me how proud he is of his family and their success with the vineyard and orchard. But underneath all this I sense that he has been anxious to get away and begin something new.

So we are perfect for each other. I can help him with all his childhood hurts. Our priest once told me that everyone carries some tough baggage through life. Mine is not as heavy as Eric's, that's for sure. As I wonder how to unload some of my extra baggage, I hear people say, "Turn it over to God!" Seems easier said than done. I just wish Eric and I could try that.

CHAPTER 6

ROBERTA

After saying goodbye to Agatha, I stared at my desk, gritted my teeth and decided to work on my ledger for the tax season. This should take my mind off so many other concerns weighing me down. Prince, my border collie, came and put his nose on my knee. I hugged him and he went over and curled up on the rug near the warm fire. It's amazing how he senses my feelings and understands me.

The phone rang. "Hi, Roberta. It's Vivian next door. I'm wondering, would you be able to give me a hand with the horses this morning? Jack is away and our critters are so restless. They hate being confined in the barn on snow days." I told her a hesitant, "Yes, I'll be over in a bit," thinking to myself, darn it, an unexpected interruption. But then, I gradually adjusted my attitude, telling myself I need to be a good neighbor.

While I was changing my clothes, the phone rang again. "Mom, I made it here to the armory. No problem." "Eric, it's so good to hear your voice. How was your trip?" "Well—the trip was okay. We're spending a couple of days here getting set to take off. Not everyone is excited about this tour, especially some of the female soldiers with families. We had a good briefing from the commander this morning. We'll do okay when we get to Afghanistan." "Honey, I miss you already, and Prince seems to know you'll be gone for awhile."

Eric then told me about some of the other soldiers (men and women) who were deploying with him and mentioned they came from all corners of the state. I sensed from Eric that he and they seemed hesitant or wary about taking over the combat hospital near Kandahar. Then I told him, "Call me before you leave. And remember our promise to pray for you every day."

"Oh, before you go…what am I supposed to do with that mysterious envelope you left on the kitchen table?" "What envelope?" he asked. "Didn't you leave a sealed envelope on the kitchen table?" He paused to think. "Is it the one that says not to open yet?" "Yes, that's it," I said. He replied, "I gave that to Jim last night and he must have forgotten it in the kitchen…you know, after all the beer we put down. Would you please see that he gets it?"

Eric promised to be in touch with me again as we said our goodbyes. So my morning ended up feeding and caring for horses at Vivian's. The taxes could wait.

CHAPTER 7

THE LETTER

Jim,

When you kicked me, for a split second there on the floor at the bar, I thought of my dad. That was the worst part.

I want you to know that I understand and forgive you.

You still are and will always be my best friend.

Alcohol killed dad. Let's not let it kill us.

Eric

CHAPTER 8

ERIC

Before leaving for the Middle East, I decided to try to get things right with Mother. When I was seven years old and we were having so much trouble with Dad, I kept wondering why she didn't protect me from him or move away with me to live somewhere else. I knew he was tormenting her, too. At night I would overhear their arguments—the shouting, things being thrown around and broken, and even her screams. That usually happened after I was in bed, and I remember hoping he would stay out of my room. I would cry myself to sleep only to wake up in the middle of a nightmare screaming. I kept dreaming that I was floating helplessly in mid-air and boulders were falling all around me and hitting me. Maybe I got those fearful dream images from my videogames. They bought me lots of videogames and told me to be quiet and stay in my room. I grew up pretty much alone.

When I was twelve, after Dad died, Aunt Agatha invited me to come and stay with her a few times. She and I had some very serious talks about our family. At first, I told her our family troubles were probably all my fault, although I couldn't exactly remember why. I felt guilty about being helpless, about running away, and about causing so much grief for my parents. She tried to make me realize what I couldn't understand as a child. She patiently explained about Dad's drinking problems and Mother's efforts to keep our family and their business together no matter what. As Dad's health became worse, all the responsibility for our vineyard and orchard fell on Mother. Aunt Agatha also told me that Mother couldn't do more than she did. Over and over I was told that our troubles were not my fault but that they would leave me with memories that probably would be very hard or impossible to forget.

As much as I try to make things better at home, I still can't make myself feel close to Mother. We get along pretty well in ordinary day-to-day ways, but there's an emotional distance between us. A year ago I pushed her out of my way in the kitchen as I was taking off to go drinking with Jim. She was trying to block me from going out and begging me not to leave. We exchanged a few cuss words. It turned into a bad scene. So that's what I needed to clear up with her before I left. I made the call and she accepted my apology, and she apologized to me for the names she called me. I'm hoping that will improve our relationship. No doubt about it, I really do love her dearly.

CHAPTER 9

ERIC

"Eric, get a move on. It's time to go." I heard that. I picked up all my stuff and hustled to the car. I'm already so far away from home in this strange part of the country. I'm not sure I even know these relatives who came to pick me up. I think I heard about them from Mother when I was a kid. But that was a long time ago. We get to their home and I wait in the living room. I don't have much time before I need to be at the airfield to catch my plane. Strange, these family friends just leave me to myself. I'm sitting here trying to remember something about them and to think about my trip.

Before long, they drop me off at a neighbor's house. It's a big place. "Eric, what time is your flight?" I try to remember. I can't remember. The exact time for my departure won't come to mind. But I know it's very soon. My ticket's in my bag. Yes, I need to find my bag right away. And so my search begins. I look for my stuff all over their house, in every room, upstairs in bedroom after bedroom, downstairs in the kitchen and in the living room, even in the basement. No bag. So, I repeat my search throughout the house again and again. Still no bag! Time is getting short. I'm worried—no, I'm desperate. I know. Maybe my bag is in the car—yes, in the car probably. I head outside.

These people live in an interesting neighborhood. Their homes are crowded together. Their streets are winding and narrow. I don't see any cars parked outside. It's midday and the air is fragrant with flowers and the sky is alive with seagulls. I see the shore at the end of the street. There's a steep path over there down through rocks to the water but I decide not to take it. I'm in such a hurry. Where's the car? I don't see any cars.

Suddenly I realize I'm lost. I can't find the street back to the house. This is so frustrating. I realize I can't even ask anyone for help. And now I don't know the name of the street and I can't remember the people's last name. Has the plane left without me? Yes, probably gone by now. I'm alone. I'm trying to start a new life. My memory won't work. I can't solve things. I can't get to where I need to be. I've never been so frustrated. What can I do?

I'm jarred awake. Oh, my God! I shake my head a few times and jump out of my bunk here at the barracks. Oh God, it was a dream! A very bad dream! So real! I hope I never again wander alone into that dream.

For just a moment, staring at my bed, I wonder what all that meant! It was such a feeling of helplessness. Awful! Hey, I've never felt like that...except, well...maybe around Dad. Then I assure myself, "I am not helpless. I am a sergeant."

CHAPTER 10

ROBERTA

"Good morning. Is this Mrs. Roberta Stevens?" "Yes…" "I'm Mrs. Tolman calling from SGLI (Soldiers' Group Life Insurance) to verify some information with you.…Are you Sergeant Eric Stevens' mother?" "Why, yes…is there something the matter?" "No, Mrs. Stevens, our reason for calling is to verify that you are Sergeant Stevens' mother and the person he designated as beneficiary for his military life insurance policy.…In the event a soldier dies, his or her beneficiary is awarded $400,000 under the policy…"

That call set me back. It was a horrible shock. I asked myself, "Could tragedy be getting closer?" A call to Agatha set me straight. She calmed my fears. We figured Eric should keep safe in the hospital, out of harm's way. But then again…

Eric's doing the work he's cut out for. In college he had good grades and wanted to major in premed. Then he considered nursing and finally graduated with the biology major. And he loved being in the Oregon National Guard during college. From teenage years, his passion for caring for people in pain drew him to them like a magnet. He was always noticing and looking out for someone who needed help at school or here at home. "Compassion" should be his middle name. Sergeant Eric Compassion Stevens! Some of the stories he writes from Afghanistan certainly show he's fully involved in the work he loves.

An early spring this year brought our trees and grapes to life back in February. I can count on it being a good year. Emilee quit her job at the grocery in town and is helping me. She's a self-starter and goes about our work without needing much supervision. I'm able to pay her a decent salary. She and I often have lunch together and I enjoy her company as well as getting to know her.

I haven't heard from Jim for awhile. Emilee tells me he's thinking about moving away from home to McMinnville near his work at The Mustang. I guess he's at that age now when he needs to be more independent. He and Agatha have had a good conversation or two. She told me that she's very concerned about him and praying for him. Apparently Agatha and Jim are hitting it off well so far. She's a gem.

All of us enjoyed having Eric home from Fort Dix last month for a few days on pass before they left for three weeks of additional theater training in Kuwait. After that they were ready to replace the medical unit serving at the hospital in Afghanistan. He was with us after spending eight weeks in New Jersey and told me it was interesting, demanding and thorough. They had medic training, many equipment checks, inspections, family information forms to complete, and lots of boxes on the checklist to complete before being deployed. God bless him. One of his first jobs was checking everyone's feet during and after long patrols. He told me he's called "Doc, the foot man."

PART TWO

Kandahar

CHAPTER 11

ERIC

Another hot April day here at the combat support hospital in Kandahar! Last night was a cool 65 degrees but today it's heading up to 100 again. Unlike Oregon, there's no rain—almost never—just dust. My first month here in this deadly scene has been tough.

All hell broke loose yesterday. Soldiers from the Sabloghay Army Camp were on foot patrol doing clearance operations in the Zari District. They got surrounded and attacked by rockets, smoke grenades and mortars near the Siah Choy and Loya Derah villages. Three men, a female soldier and two old Afghan civilians were brought in on the Black Hawk helicopter. My first job was to check them out when they arrived—scan them for weapons, ammunition, and grenades before bringing them into the hospital. In the emergency area, I worked with their blast injuries, some severe bleeding and a few penetrating chest injuries. One soldier had his hand practically blown off by a smoke grenade.

I cleaned his wounds and stabilized him before we shipped him north on the Black Hawk to the Bagram Airfield Hospital near Kabul. There's a hand surgeon up there who'll treat him. We never know what's going to hit us next.

One of my buddies asked, "Eric, when are you going to get promoted from combat medic to a doc?" My job's about basic survival. I take care of combat injuries and stabilize people until we get more help. I know it's going to take some time to get me more certified. I'm already doing almost everything our nursing staff does. My job at the hospital also takes me out into the field to deal with emergencies. I'm still feeling like a beginner but with a ton of experience. Soldiers call me "Doc," even though I'm not a full doctor.

Our hospital is a Level 3 combat support hospital. We have a pharmacy, lab and x-ray, an intensive care unit, internal care wards, and the emergency unit where I work. My supervisor is Major Jose Rodriguez. He's a nurse who's served in the National Guard for 25 years. At home he has a wife and three children. In a lot of ways, he is like a dad to us, physicians and nurses included. I've worked out some of my stuff with him. He's a man you can go to for just about anything. The others here feel the same. He's good at dealing with fear and confusion. He's really smart, supportive and a great leader. We're lucky to have him here.

When I first got here we had two injured Taliban insurgents in our ward. These guys were tough to care for. I got spit at, cursed and hit once. Same for our nurses. Surprisingly, both these guys spoke fluent English. That was tough—caring for terrorists along with everyone else. But that's Army policy. All injured in combat are cared for in assigned places at our hospital including our military, civilians and even enemies. Major Rodriguez helped me deal with some anger about that.

CHAPTER 12

ERIC

Army Sergeant Clark Kenton came here on the Medevac helicopter about a week ago. Kenton was wounded on mission when his vehicle got blasted by an IED (improvised explosive device) on a road to Kandahar. He, a buddy and their Humvee were sent flying and on fire into a ditch where he emerged with three broken ribs, a crushed knee, and shrapnel. He nearly lost his left leg. We can't remove the shrapnel between his shoulders and neck here in our hospital.

I've become friends with Sergeant Kenton, and he's been filling me in about combat. This is his seventh deployment. "Eric," he said, "There's nothing as exciting as fighting for your life, killing before getting killed." I asked him, "What mindset makes that possible?" He replied, "There's a mantra I've needed to repeat over and over in my mind: 'Soldier, that's the way it is. Drive on.'" He told me that fear is his worst enemy. "You mask your fear because fear is contagious.

So rather than fear, you show anger...the on-switch gets thrown and you're like a racecar in the red....The people you're with get killed. We never know who'll be next. You want to settle the score by taking enemy lives, but the score can never really be settled. So it's easier to kill them." Then he explained about shooting to kill and how to overcome that natural human fear.

"In Iraq I killed almost a hundred people. I had pictures of them on my digital camera. On leave, I showed them to my wife back home. I watched her eyes. First, I could see fear. Then terror. I deleted those trophy pictures. She has a tough time reconciling my deployment to Afghanistan. She thinks I should get some mental health care....But I can't afford the 'damaged goods' label in my career."

The next day, I was able to get into a conversation about mental health with him. He finds it okay to confide in me. What he told me sounds like PTSD (post traumatic stress disorder). "Eric," Sgt. Kenton said, "I have panic attacks and nightmares you wouldn't believe. This has been going on for almost a year. I'm grateful that I'm getting meds for pain and sleep. I do feel secluded here, and that's like before when I lost interest in others." I tell him he's safe here. "Well, most of the time, but I'm always on guard, checking for threats. Being here slows me down. I need conflict to feel alive."

I asked Clark about his greatest fear. "To die alone," he said. And your greatest hopes? "I want to be like a warm stone getting polished. I want to see my children and grandchildren. I want to be a good husband and father to my three children." He smiled at me. Tears came to his eyes. "Oh," he whispered, "I told this to the chaplain. Ever since I came to the hospital, I'm experiencing prayer. It's not like anything I've felt before. I can feel this deep inside, and I know it's there. It's like God is close to me—and that's all the time, day and night."

CHAPTER 13

ERIC

Yesterday Nadia, a young Afghan mother who lives nearby, brought her eight-year-old son Masoud to us. He had a high fever and was dizzy. Security at our entrance paged me. As the mother's eyes met mine, they beseeched me...desperately begging help. She spoke no English but I understood. I got down on my knees and reached for her boy. Masoud stumbled back, afraid. My smile began to solve that. I put my hand on his forehead and felt his fever. He stared at me. His eyes reminded me of a deer's eyes in the headlights. Then, as he collapsed, I caught him.

We carried him into our emergency room. But first, we had to wand both mother and son for weapons. Nadia's soft, devout words begging Allah's help accompanied us into the hospital. The boy's blood pressure was very low and he was severely dehydrated. We injected him with antibiotics and put him on an IV. After the doctor finished checking him, we found a little space for the boy and his mother near the nursing desk. Fortunately, Masoud's fever lifted overnight and he was well enough to return home. Through our interpreter I assured Nadia that I would check Masoud again in a week. A grateful mother with her son and a pack of antibiotics departed from us smiling.

I've been doing some thinking at night about Sergeant Kenton and prayer. I ask myself, do I really pray? I do, especially when I'm cleansing wounds and working on sore feet. My prayer, like that of the Afghan mother, is about wanting help. I also pray that I can stay calm and deescalate high-powered fears in wounded soldiers. One of our nurses got this practice across to me. She's very good with people and a good teacher.

Our health care specialist here in the hospital is very efficient. She accomplishes about twice as much as I do. But, she also seems abrupt with patients and staff. I wonder about that. Her conversations with me stay cordial, to the point and brief. She has been deployed at least four times and served in several combat support hospitals in Iraq and Afghanistan with Major Rodriguez. In these combat support hospitals we deal with so many casualties and such hardship, it's no wonder some of us need to become emotionally distant.

My medic work also tears me apart sometimes. I never imagined the suffering some of our soldiers endure. It's not only physical—it's mental and emotional, too. Just touching people in pain gives me a different feel. Touching wounds outside and inside…I know some of these will be healed but many remain scars for life in a world that turns unfamiliar and dangerous. I try my best. But I know when we finish with our care the end result is not up to us.

CHAPTER 14

MAJOR JOSE RODRIGUEZ

This morning Sergeant Eric Stevens accompanied twenty Army Soldiers on a search patrol to a village about two miles downrange. His medic duty was to monitor for heat fatigue and deal with combat injuries if necessary. Ordinarily these platoon search missions along that road have been relatively safe and without incident. Today was tragically different.

Mortar fire, rockets and grenades flew at them from all directions. The ambush killed or wounded nearly all the men and destroyed all but one Humvee. We lost four soldiers, while thirteen wounded were rescued and brought here, filling our ICU and wards. Our fallen soldiers, along with the three most critically injured, were transported to Bagram. We are short of help. No time off. No breaks. This is my first chance—at midnight—to record the day's incidents in this personal journal.

Remarkably, our Sergeant Stevens escaped physical harm. Here is the brief account he gave me:

"Two other soldiers and I turned out to be the only ones not physically wounded. All of us probably suffered concussions from the blast. For a moment everything went black for me. When I came to, I tried to figure out what was happening—then did. Our Humvee door wouldn't close. The vehicle in front of us was on fire. I grabbed the fire extinguisher and ran to the burning Humvee. Then I snapped to, realizing my duty was to save guys. I pulled two men away from their vehicle and got some help from another soldier. It felt like a dream—no time, terrifying silence after the blast was over. We hid beside the road. I reached for my cell phone and called. I remember lots of blood. I held Soldier Adams as he was dying. He asked me if he was dying. I didn't know what to say. He called out for his mother, then gasped, and stopped breathing. I don't remember much more."

I take great pride in my staff. We've spent this entire day and night keeping a number of soldiers alive while we and they grieve their dead and wounded buddies. Today, ours is a mixture of great sadness and urgent hope. Finally, young Sgt. Eric Stevens is a hero in our midst.

CHAPTER 15

ERIC

I stayed on the scene until all wounded men were transported. Once I came to my senses, I remember being in high gear. God, it was awful. I needed to think. I needed to make sure everyone was taken care of. Thinking was taking all my strength. I kept closing my eyes and gritting my teeth to make me concentrate. I helped with the rescue. I repeated over and over, I've got to get these guys out of here. I lifted some of them off the ground and carried them to our John Deere Gator. I had no idea what time it was. It didn't matter. Then I was among the last to be taken back to our hospital.

One of our nurses descended on me and made me sit down on a chair in the emergency room. They were working on four soldiers. Quiet confusion reigned. They needed help. I could see that. I started to move. Our nurse looked at me and gave a firm, "No. Stay put." I was annoyed…restless…agitated…angry. Then the attending physician came over and checked me. He sent me to my bunk for enforced rest. No arguments allowed. I can't stand keeping still. Well, so much for me!

I had a concussion but it only took a few hours to recover except for the ringing in my ears. Other soldiers had nasty problems at night trying to sleep and poor concentration or memory lapses during the day. But I was spared these symptoms and told to avoid alcohol or drugs, neither of which I have used since being deployed.

The memory of that horrendous scene keeps coming back to me...haunting me. Men dying. The young soldier begging for his mother. Excruciating suffering. So much bleeding. Soldiers really scared. The close call on my life. But I made it. Why me? Why am I so lucky?

Major Rodriguez and I talked this through. He assured me that I am fit for duty. So now I have to lock those haunting memories away in a mental safe and endeavor to forget about them. I'll always remember his advice: "Eric, you don't get over it; you get on with it."

CHAPTER 16

EMILEE

It's been awhile since Eric wrote, and his letters take ages to get here. This time he told me about Nadia and Masoud, the Afghan mother and boy they cared for several weeks ago. He told me he and the interpreter went by their home to check on Masoud but the boy was at school, which is a good thing. Nadia also has two younger children who were at home. Apparently, her husband is away doing police training. It sounds to me like this family likes Eric—and they should, after all he did for them. He asked me to shop for a book with lots of pictures of America to give to the family. Anyway, I'm glad Eric is getting to know some of the people there. I'm sure he'll have a few good stories to tell when he gets home.

Working for Roberta the Winegrower is going well. I'm learning a lot about vineyards and their care. Right now we're doing the early spring routine. I've been spreading pumice compost, which is very light and porous, to improve the quality and water-holding capability of the topsoil around our vines. It's time consuming but it keeps me outside. which I love. My next project will be checking out the drip irrigation system, and to install a new one in the vineyard that was just planted. We're going to add bacterial and fungal microbes to the irrigation system as fertilizers. Roberta told me our goal with the organic microbe fertilizers is to create self-nourishing soils. After that, she is going to teach me how to prepare mildew sprays that use special oils, and we'll also plant some native grasses to deal with pest management. I'm impressed by her knowledge and skills. I'm glad to have this job.

Sometimes I worry about Roberta. I know it must be hard for her to be living alone now. She hints at that now and then. I think having her faithful dog Prince helps. But she needs someone to talk to. We do talk at lunchtime, and that seems to cheer her up. I think she enjoys my company and that's a good sign for a future mother-in-law.

Eric also wrote me about the horrible incident while he was on patrol. He asked me not to tell Roberta about it. She might panic. He said he recovered from the blast quickly, and it only took a few hours to get rid of his headache and the ringing in his ears. Right away they cleared him as fit for duty. He told me how upset he is about the loss of those soldiers. He said he even dreams about it, especially holding the man who was dying. I will be extremely glad when he gets home. I'm counting the months. I can't wait until I'm counting the days!

CHAPTER 17

MAJOR JOSE RODRIGUEZ

I just received a letter from Army Sergeant Parker whom we cared for 18 months ago. He served with Special Operations and was critically injured during a search mission in a village not far from here. I went back and reviewed my journal account of that alarming event.

"Major, in a room in the village I encountered a Taliban commander who turned out to be a suicide bomber. With my left arm, I got the guy around his neck to choke him. He detonated his bomb and blew my right side to pieces. He died a few steps away. I knew I was dying...in thick smoke, bleeding profusely. My brain kept telling my lungs: keep breathing, keep breathing. I feared I was going to Hell. I reached out to God. I've made 100 promises to God that I haven't kept. On the spot I said, 'God, if you will look into my heart right now you will see that it is more sincere than ever before. If you spare my life, I will serve you the way you wanted me to.'

"Immediately—a miracle I think—my guys showed up. They came out of nowhere into the room and worked on me. They put a tourniquet on my groin to stop the bleeding but couldn't do that around my shoulder. They tied my arm to my body, hoping that would slow the bleeding. They brought me here to the hospital. All the guys in my unit and some Navy Seals gave blood to save me. I remember you told me this amounted to 36 units of blood and 12 units of plasma."

As a result of this incident, Sergeant Parker has had 20 surgeries in the United States. And he tells me he's in good physical health. His wife jokingly tells him that when he's naked his right side looks like a patchwork quilt. A critical decision was whether or not to amputate his disabled right arm. Physicians put the burden of choice on him. He resolved to keep his arm and that meant a series of surgeries transplanting tendons from his wrist and arm to his hand to enable him to grip and use his fingers.

In his letter, he tells me that he has his physical self under control; the next step is his mental and emotional agenda. He writes: "I suffer especially with anger and strong feelings of hate. I break out in a sweat when these feelings intrude. Then I think, 'I'll get in trouble if I do that.' I tell myself, every action has a consequence and I don't want to end up in jail. I keep dreaming that I'm stuck in that room, rethinking how to get out, how to escape, or a way to do it differently. I find it hard to trust. But, most of all, I have a hard time distinguishing between work and home. I act like a sergeant in both places. Frankly, my wife, my kids and our dog are afraid of me because I unintentionally lose it. My wife is so loving and understanding, and she's made it very clear to me that I'm messed up in the head. So, my next step is treatment for PTSD. Major, please keep us in your prayers."

CHAPTER 18

JIM

Last month when I showed up for work at The Mustang the boss told me we were going to have a conversation in the back room. That seemed strange. When we went back there, I was astonished to see my parents, Sister Agatha and a counselor whom I had not met. Down deep I immediately sensed what this was about. I was right. It was an intervention.

My Dad opened the meeting assuring me that he and Mom love me dearly but can't bear to see me waste my life the way I'm doing with alcohol. He brought up the nasty arguments we've been having at home and how I isolate myself from everyone. Mom spoke to me about the changes she's noticed in me and a lot of her worries. Sister Agatha didn't share anything I told her in confidence, but urged me to cooperate and get help to deal with what she called "an addiction." The boss backed her up, mentioning the times I didn't show up for work or got drunk on my shift and was out of control. He said, "Go to treatment and keep your job. Otherwise, you're out of here. Find work somewhere else." The counselor told me to take every word they said seriously.

It all seemed to happen so fast. My first reaction was escape. Balk. That quickly turned into shame. Then regret. Clearly, everyone had had enough of me. Do I give in to all these people who love and respect me? Can I change? Is it even possible? This is out of my hands. I agreed to get help sometime soon. Surprisingly, the counselor told me that they are ready for me now at the recovery center. Mom brought my suitcase packed with clothes. The boss shook my hand and wished me luck. Before I knew it, I was in the car with the counselor and on my way.

In recovery, I began working the 12 steps. The first three about powerlessness took a long time and a lot of introspection and prayer. I realized that, at first, I used to worry about how my drinking would affect my work and home life. But, after Eric left, that began to change. I drank more to stop guilt, sweats and shakes. I was edgy and reeked. And then I started worrying about work or home interfering with my drinking. Sister Agatha spotted that change and talked with me about it long before our intervention. I think she's the one to thank for getting me into recovery.

I've confronted my anger habit, too. Anger is a

show of strength? Wrong. To forgive and to love, that's strength. That's what I'm working on now.

I'm back on the job. I get to AA meetings. I'm taking one day at a time. Most of all, I'm grateful to everyone who had the guts to be at that intervention. They mean a lot to me. I love them and always will.

CHAPTER 19

ERIC

This month we are halfway into our deployment here. Afghanistan's summer heat bears down on us and they tell us that the hot season should bring quieter days and nights. Not so far. Last night someone sprayed DEATH TO FOREIGN OCCUPIERS on our outside wall. The spelling was perfect, and one of our nurses is convinced the perpetrator is one of the troublesome insurgents we took in and cared for last winter.

I have lost track of the number of patients we've treated since we arrived here. Serving with this highly professional Oregon National Guard Medical Unit is an honor. These men and women are totally dedicated to our mission, and they work tirelessly to provide the best possible medical care. I'm wondering if I should make a career of military medical service...perhaps under less stressful circumstances.

Day after day I think of the time we were wiped out on patrol and how I might have been more capable and saved more lives. Often at night I have painful nightmares about that patrol. Guilt about the man that I held as he died still haunts me. Many other details of that day escape me. What always sticks with me is the terrible anguish the young soldier and I experienced as he died in my arms. This memory is my toughest inner struggle. I wish I could visit his mother in Arkansas to tell her about his very last word…Mother.

Major Rodriguez and I talked about my state of mind again today. I can't remember meeting a man who is so understanding and willing to help. He is getting me to recall and repeat the story of the ambush. I have been battling those memories and trying to put them out of my mind, especially when I'm working in the emergency room. But they never go away, especially at night. During our meetings, Major asks me to close my eyes and unlock the place where I store my most fearsome memories. Then I describe this traumatic scene to him with all the detail and feeling I can muster. He also records this conversation for me to listen to later. It's not easy to listen to my voice, but I man-up and do it. This combat stress therapy seems to help.

I've met a few times before with the Major. Today a few more details came out and I felt less uptight and guilty. With him I'm unlocking sealed-up terror, defusing it and letting it become more a part of me and my story rather than keeping it in a cage where it secretly gnaws away at me incessantly. I think I feel less troubled, guilty, haunted. And, I'm beginning to sleep better. I'm not there yet, but I'm working on it. It feels right.

CHAPTER 20

AGATHA

I am so pleased that Jim agreed to address his problem with substance abuse. He is a fine young man with a promising life ahead of him. He and I have spoken about his anger habit. He thinks anger was his best source of strength and most effective weapon to avoid being bullied. In treatment he learned that strength is found in forgiveness and love, and that is always challenging. I sent a letter to Eric about Jim being in the recovery program and asked his prayers for Jim. Eric doesn't write often, but this time he answered me practically by return mail. He promised his prayers.

Eric writes the ambush over there was so brutal that during the nights following his concussion he has been thinking more about God. He also mentioned the St. Joseph medal we gave him. He thinks St. Joseph must be helping him care for all those injured people. He wrote: "Aunt Agatha, I'm keeping my prayer and faith very simple. For me it is about trust. Joseph cared for Mary and Jesus. He was a good father and a good model. I'm looking forward to being a good father someday."

Tucked in his letter is a picture of a Pashtun mother with her boy. On the back he wrote, "Wonderful people, Nadia and Masoud, whom we cared for awhile back. They bring me fresh baked bread, a real treat." He said he added their photo to the little picture album we gave him before he left. I don't think he understands their Pashto language but that doesn't stand in the way of their friendship. In some ways, I think, they are like a family away from home to him.

With the rise of the Taliban, women's rights have been more restricted, so Nadia and her children live in relative seclusion. However, Eric's interpreter told him Nadia is an educated woman who writes poetry, and she is a possible candidate to become the village Qaryadar someday. (I had to look that title up in my encyclopedia!) A Qaryadar is the female village leader who, among other duties, arranges for religious festivals, arbitrates conflicts between men and women, and prepares deceased females for burial and performs final services for them.

During these past months, I have grown to appreciate the service our medical men and women provide in such perilous circumstances. And I think a great deal about the people living and raising families in countries torn apart by war. All my life I have prayed for peace in the world. I continue to hope for the time when we will experience peace and understanding, not only among peoples of the world, but also among our friends and members of our own families. Maybe that kind of burning hope within me helps me stay peaceful. If only—with hope—we could encourage everyone in the world to pray for peace and to be peacemakers!

CHAPTER 21

ERIC

Wounded soldiers are everywhere in our emergency room. More are crowding in. Where is the staff? I can't see them. How can I manage this alone? Distorted faces glide by, one after another in pain—their eyes begging.

BOOM!

What? What was that? Was I dreaming? Wait. An explosion? I jump from bed. Where? I throw on a shirt and pull my pants on.

A huge fire rages down the road. It's one of the houses down there. Screams break through the darkness. Shadows move on the road. Oh God, someone's been bombed. Wailing pierces the smoky night air. People are running here. We are on full alert. From the shadows a man brings a child in his arms. A woman screams. Oh no…It's Masoud. The boy is limp in his father's arms, scarcely breathing. We place him on the stretcher and carry him inside. The father is crying and hitting his head with both hands. Masoud seems to be dying. More people come running to our hospital. I look down at my bare feet. They are covered with blood.

We do all we can to save Masoud. But we fail. He dies. Now Masoud's father tells us that Nadia and the other younger children have also died in the explosion. He weeps. He is hysterical—a father who has suddenly lost everyone and everything. Our gentle nurse takes care of him. He wants to return to his destroyed home and his loved ones lying dead in the ashes. She accompanies him back down the dark road.

Tears come to my eyes. Long ago I resolved not to cry, no matter what. But I can't help it. Knowing that in an instant a family is torn to pieces…the human savagery overwhelms me. And they are kind people, people I love.

Sitting here beside Masoud's body, I wonder if this horrible tragedy is my fault. Could this have happened because I am their American friend? Did the insurgents see us speaking to one another with our interpreter? Walking together? Being friends? Oh God, forgive me. I can't bear this. I bow my head and try to stop thinking.

CHAPTER 22

MAJOR JOSE RODRIGUEZ

Following the loss of the Afghan family, Sergeant Eric Stevens experienced severe nightmares, more night sweats, grief and hypertension. While he continued to perform fairly well, I worried about his mental health. Often his remarks on duty were inappropriate, and he tended to isolate himself from the staff. I kept meeting with him and provided what counsel and support I could. But I was not optimistic about any immediate improvement in his condition.

My care for Eric came to an end a month later. One of our physicians and I went to the 10 km. race at the Kandahar Airfield. We weren't running. We assisted with any possible injuries. On the return trip—just a hundred yards or so from our combat support hospital—a youngster was sprawled out on the side of the road. We stopped to check on him. Immediately we were fired upon as the youngster got up and ran away.

I was wounded in my lower leg, in the femoral artery in my groin, and with shrapnel in my upper arm. Our physician collapsed onto the road from her wounds.

The saying is true: "You never hear the one that hits you." I was dazed. Everything went into slow motion. I was losing it. I said to myself, "I have to get down"—but I couldn't react. Then I looked at my leg spurting blood. I jammed my thumb into the leg wound. I heard the last round—BAM—then all was silent. I heard birds chirping. I was mad as hell because then they kept firing. I saw a hose of blood shooting from my groin. I pinched my femoral artery to stop the bleeding there and from my leg. Guards from the hospital started firing back as they came running to us. The physician with me was probably dead, and she did die. I sat by her until they came with the Gator, first to take her and then return for me. Someone stayed to help me. I was sure I was dying, too. I passed out.

I guess God has more for me to do, I thought, when I woke up in our ICU. I looked over to my left. Eric was sitting beside my bed watching me with a frozen stare. He continued to keep vigil by me practically day and night. Another medic stepped up and took over Eric's regular duties in the emergency unit.

In a few days I was transferred to the Bagram Airfield Hospital near Kabul and then to the hospital in Germany.

Our commander approved Eric's request to accompany me on this journey. He cared for me like a faithful son and attentive medic all along the way. He even stayed with me in Germany while he received some psychiatric help. He was sent home to the States a few weeks before I was able to return to Oregon.

The National Guard sent three temporary replacements to our combat support hospital: a physician, a combat medic and a nurse. The work of life saving for all injured continues there. The flag in our hearts flies at half-staff.

PART THREE

Homecoming

CHAPTER 23

EMILEE

Eric's been home for a week. We're not sure for how long. He tells me he's itching to re-deploy and finish his service with the medical team. I hadn't even gotten to the point where I was counting the days for his home-coming! And here he is, home a few months early.

Eric's looking good. I wasn't sure what to expect after hearing about the ambush and his concussion. But, he's sort of upbeat, really glad to see me, and he seems happy to be home. He's very quiet, a bit edgy, and not much for conversation.

I wanted to give Eric a big party at my place and invite all my friends, but he begged me not to go to the trouble. He said he'd like to kick back for awhile and enjoy keeping things simple. But, you know Roberta! No one was going to talk her out of a welcome-home celebration for Eric. So, the day after he came home the American flag went up in her dining room, very special wines and beers emerged from the cellar, and I put up a banner for him: JOB WELL DONE.

Roberta and I cooked while Eric watched TV up in his room that evening. There were just the five of us at her place that night. Aunt Agatha and Jim arrived together. He picked her up in Portland. Agatha gave Eric a big kiss and Jim gave him a bear hug. It was beautiful watching their reunion. Not much was said between them, but you sure could feel their love.

Roberta obviously knew what happened to Eric in Afghanistan. She's been watching him like a hawk. He plays it cool with her. She asks him how he is, how he feels. His response is always "great." I know she suspects he's fibbing, but she doesn't force anything more out of him. I warned her about that.

During our times alone, Eric told me more about the hospital in Kandahar and their traumatic experiences. Hearing about all that human damage gave me the creeps.

This week, when he's not going to Portland for therapy, he helps in the orchard. He just goes to work and doesn't have much to say. He likes to keep busy. The other day somebody moved his stuff. He got raging mad and left for awhile. After that, he was okay. It doesn't take much to set him off. I hope he'll be less up-tight when he gets more distance from Afghanistan. I keep trying to help him be mellow.

CHAPTER 24

JIM

At Roberta's, Eric told me we need to get together. "Jim, I need a break. Let's take a day and night off from all this stress. I want to hit the bar. We need to talk. Okay?" I told him to meet me at The Mustang and then after work we'll go over to my new place in McMinnville. Eric knows I'm not into alcohol anymore, and he says that's okay. But I thought there'd be tension over that. We might not hit it off the way we used to. That's what I first thought.

Eric's been a hero to me since he deployed. I was planning to tell him about my intervention and treatment program…hoping to get some ideas and encouragement from him. But the opposite happened. He's needy. He's leaning on me more than ever for support. He tells me he's drinking to forget the horrible memories he brought with him from Afghanistan.

After I finished my shift at 2:00 a.m. and he put down several beers, we headed to my place. All night our conversation was easy but also intense. No doubt about it, we're still best friends. He told me a few hair-raising stories about his work at the hospital. But he really wanted to tell me about how hard it is to be home and how tough it is to get a night's sleep. He's getting along okay with Roberta and Emilee. That's not the issue right now. It's about waking up halfway through the night, revved up, and then dealing with nightmares and night sweats until morning.

"I guess my problem," he told me, "is that there's no one around for me to help or take care of. So, I feel lonely…very lonely…useless…disgusted with myself. I started drinking to push all that out of my mind. It works for me, Jim, but only for half a night. I feel like I'm haunted. Does that sound sick?" I shook my head, "No, not sick, Eric."

"Alcohol calmed my night problems for a few hours at night, but when it wore off I'd light up like a Christmas tree, sit up in bed and stay awake for hours on end. As I tried to go back to sleep, that's when bad dreams would hassle me."

We talked on and on into the morning. Not much sleep! Eric told me he's going for therapy and they are talking about a medication that could help him with sleep and nightmares, but he needs to quit or cut back on the drinking. I think he can. I also told him about what I learned in my recovery program: "Let go and let God." I need to face life as it is, forgive myself and love myself. That's like the idea Sister Agatha gave me: "You are okay to be the man you are. God doesn't bless frauds!"

We stayed up all night…sharing at a deep level. As it got to be morning we ended up laughing about all the stupid stuff we did in high school. It was a night I'll never forget.

CHAPTER 25

ERIC

I was over in Hell for eight months. But I had a job. I worked my butt off taking care of wounded men, women and children. Some of them didn't make it. "Try to forget Hell," I tell myself. "That's the way it is; move on." Not convincing. Stop thinking about anything but work. Forget moaning over why we are there. Forget about what's going on at home. Forget about how I feel. Keep working. Focus. Focus.

Over there, I even forgot what Mom, Emilee, Jim and Aunt Agatha looked like. That was terrible. I tried to picture them in my mind. Their faces wouldn't come to me. Over and over I'd reach for the little picture album they gave me to remind me. But time stands still in pictures.

Some nights, I tried to think about Prince. He's such a good dog. He used to sleep on my bed. I pretended he was there with me. Now he's confused by me. So is everyone else—except Jim. I'm trying to be like I used to be before I went away. It's damn hard to fake it. Mom especially sees through all this. I'm not doing a good job hiding from her even when I try hard. I'm not the same guy. I hate this.

Back there I started sharing a lot of deep pain with Major Rodriguez. God, I miss him. I'm trying to get help from my therapist in Portland. But it's not the same. He hasn't been in combat—he doesn't really know what it's like to have blood all over you, to hold people dying in your arms, to be knocked senseless by an IED. I'm not sure how much to tell him. Some stuff is too painful to bear when it gets released into my mind from my hidden inner self.

I know I'm wounded. No, maybe not wounded—scarred is a better word. These are scars that never go away—scars in the deepest part of myself that get between me and the people I love, even our dog Prince. I hate this.

CHAPTER 26

ROBERTA

With my son home, I feel like I'm walking on egg shells. I forgot that I changed some of the furniture in his room while he was away. So the day after he came home we had a major blow-up over that. He screamed at me. Some awful memories of his dad came to my mind.

I'm not sure how to relate to Eric. He's distant. I love him dearly and he knows that, but I can't get close to him. In these last few years I relied on his emotional support; now it's missing. Rather than getting along, we argue.

I told him, "You are creating a lot of tension around here. You should shape up." That didn't go over well! He wouldn't speak to me for the rest of the day. Agatha gave me a good idea to try. She is reading an excellent book, *Once a Warrior—Always a Warrior*, by Col. Charles Hoge, MD. His advice, she said, is to stop using "You" and "should" statements with Eric. So that night I told him, "Honey, this morning I meant to say, "*I'm* feeling a lot of tension here. Maybe *we* can make things better."

He stared at me and then seemed to melt. I could see it in his eyes. He blinked a few times, lowered his head, thought a minute and then looked up at me. His instinct to care about others was kicking in and, believe it or not, he came over and gave me a hug and apologized. Amazing how language can make such a difference in relationships!

Now that we are making small break-throughs at home, I sense we could do better. I know this will take time and tons of patience for both of us. I'm sharing my hopes about our business with him, and getting him to share his ideas with me. While he was in Afghanistan I kept my problems to myself, and he spared me all the grief he experienced over there. We no longer counted on one another.

Time drifted away. Both of us changed. While I suffer privately, I'm resolved to pray for Eric and for us. I need to stay strong, to be honest with him, to watch my words, and not nag.

CHAPTER 27

ERIC

"His name is Jason Newmark. He's your age. Like you, he's a sergeant." My therapist, Dr. Keller, had something up his sleeve, an unexpected surprise. He coaxed me to consider giving Jason a temporary job at our vineyard, and putting him up until he gets his own place. I thought a moment, and then asked, "Do you really think I'm up to helping him? That this could work?"

Jason lost his lower leg in Iraq awhile back, made it through months of rehab with his new prosthesis, and now is ready to set out on his own. Jason's marriage is heading to a divorce and he has no family to return to. Unfortunately, he attempted suicide but is beyond that now, thanks to the medical team at the VA Hospital. Major Rodriguez, a friend of my therapist, apparently called and suggested I'd be the ideal guy to help Jason with his next steps. I guess Jason was one of Major Rodriguez's patients in Iraq.

Dr. Keller explained this would not only be good for Jason, but for me, too. I owned up to feeling and being reclusive and hard to get along with at home. He already spotted that. No big revelation. Now I'll be faced with relating to yet another person. Then I wondered out loud how Mom would cope with another casualty in the house.

"Eric, think about this. It's time for you to start getting out of your shell." I responded, "Inside the shell my inner self feels far away, cold—sometimes like ice." That led to our conversation about the need for more human warmth in there. My knee-jerk reaction is to back away and hide because I feel so damn guilty about the way I am. It's tough to let anyone close to me, although Mom has put a few cracks in my shell. But, that's not making much difference. I'm not into displaying my scars. They're ugly and they hurt like Hell.

"Eric, think about the possibility of working with Jason. You're both military, both the same rank, both the same age, both with a lot of pain in your lives, and both friends of Major Rodriguez. You guys could understand one another and hash things over. This would be healthy for both of you."

I told Dr. Keller I'd like to meet Jason before we make any decisions and, most of all, run this by Mom. That's how our session ended.

CHAPTER 28

AGATHA

Roberta called yesterday. "Agatha, something's come up! Eric just told me he wants to bring a wounded sergeant from Iraq here to take a job and stay at our place. I wonder how that will work. I'm not opposed, but hope Eric will be able to carry his own weight in this. Do you think I can depend on him?" I thought a moment and replied, "I think you can, but ask Eric to stop by to see me tomorrow when he's in Portland. I'd like to talk to him about this. Besides, maybe he'd be willing to meet with a class here at the college and tell them about his military experience." After our call Eric arrived and I enjoyed the rest of the afternoon with him.

Eric did a good job with one of our classes. His combat medic stories were a great hit. Then he and I sat down and talked about anger. I think this came up because Jim told him about the help I gave him with his anger habit.

Here is a brief account of my conversation with Eric today. I asked him about his experience of anger, especially when it happens and how it gets triggered. He gave me the following example: "Aunt Agatha, I picture Masoud's death, sitting there beside him in the emergency room....Just the picture in my mind triggers my anger before I even start thinking about it—out-of-control—and along with this feeling comes terrible guilt and sorrow. This happens with a lot of other casualties, too.

"Sometimes when things don't go right at home or work, I'm mad before I even think about it. I tell myself I shouldn't feel this way, but it's too late, I already do. And, that's the way my brain works. Anger comes from down deep in my memory—from out-of-reach places—where there are wounds from so much in my life that resist getting fixed."

I talked with him about using "I" statements when he got angry. For example, when Roberta changed the furniture in his room, why not first cool off and then say something like, "I got upset about the way my room looks...but I'll fix it back the way it was. No big deal," and then apologize.

Thanks to the help he got from Major Rodriguez, Eric doesn't blame others for the way he feels. He's owning his own feelings, working at not criticizing or finding fault, and trying to let resentments go. He's beginning to see the difference between "automatic emotions" that spontaneously arise from his memories or images on TV and thought-out ideas when he's making a judgment about how to act or not act. Still, lots of times these get tangled together.

Bottom line, we agreed, all is not okay just because he's now at home. And, we'll keep honoring this truth. I think this is about the cross Eric carries and manages daily, hopefully with God's help. The Cross of Christ in life may indeed absorb some pain from human suffering. But Eric's cross is there to stay—like a scar deep within him.

CHAPTER 29

ERIC

Jason and I met at the hospital where I go for therapy. He's a friendly guy. In Iraq he was hit by an IED and lost his lower leg. He's proud about the way he's getting around with his new leg. He showed me his other wounds—all of them—and then told me about his break-up with his wife. They were married only a short time before he deployed. She was lonely and found a new boyfriend while he was away. She told him she couldn't cope with him as injured. They had angry words. He said he got abusive with her, unfortunately. And, she refused to give marriage counseling a try, at least for now.

Jason's frustrated over this, blames himself, and thinks of himself as unattractive. He doesn't trust his wife and knows the feeling's mutual. So, when he comes to live with us, I have my work cut out for me. I sense I can be a buddy, and hopefully he will be able to understand my own vulnerabilities, too.

Speaking of being vulnerable, here's where I stand. (And, this is hard to put into words.) First of all, the fact that I didn't come home the same man is not intentional. No way would I intend to have these wounds that won't heal affect me and everybody else.

Probably worst of all is that my *feelings* of love for Emilee, Mom and everyone else are not there or as strong as they used to be. I haven't figured out how to change that, try as I might. There's no reason I can think of to explain this. It's just plain tough not to feel the love for them I used to feel. I care. I know they care. They love me and are trying so hard.

At first, getting to sleep and waking up in the middle of the night were big problems for me. The meds I have for sleeping help immensely. But now and then I have terrible nightmares, and the other night I threw up in my sleep. Thank God, that doesn't happen very often. I've always had vivid dreams but, since Afghanistan, they seem more life-like—so real and so horrible.

Without any notice, my combat medic experiences and even some bad stuff from growing up pop into my mind. Some tiny thing, like a familiar sound on the road or an odor at the hospital, can trigger these memories—some of them long ago forgotten. They are such a mysterious part of who I am. These memories bring anger, fear, and sometimes powerful feelings of helplessness. When I'm with others, I'm fairly good at

pretending nothing's wrong—at least I think so. That's
not always easy to do. I'm sure at times I seem to them
to be distracted, not-there, out of reach. I'm trying not
to kick myself around about this.

I guess my final vulnerability is not being clear
about where I'm going in the future. Should Emilee and
I marry? Should I be an EMT? Redeploy? Get a nursing
degree? Help Mom by taking over the business? I think
I need to find myself before I can get better.

CHAPTER 30

EMILEE

When Jason arrived a few days ago, Roberta asked him to work with me in our vineyard and orchard. He's a good worker and handy with all the machinery. With me Jason is casual, playful and talks a lot about his marriage. Nothing about that marriage sounds promising. There's a lot of hurt there. He's doing fine physically but I'm keeping him on the ground, off ladders. It's interesting working now with two sergeants. They don't talk much in front of me but I can tell they're becoming buddies.

Speaking of marriage, my desires are changing. I know Eric's not ready to take the step. At least that's what I'm sensing. When I hint how we might try to live together, he changes the subject. And, if we did move in together, I'm not sure if it would really work.

I wish we could go back to what we had. It's so sad, and the life we dreamed of doesn't seem real anymore.

Fall is here and the growing season is winding down. We still have a lot of work before winter sets in. I suspect my job will end sometime after Christmas and I'll be back inside at the grocery business. I now know the vineyard business well enough to take it over if Roberta needs me to. We're working well together. Right now Eric's doing a good job with the accounts, helping our workers, and taking care of the orchard. I have no idea what he'll do in the future. But, I know he didn't used to be serious about making this his life's work.

As for me, I'm trying to be helpful and brave about this...so far.

CHAPTER 31

ROBERTA

Now that most of our produce is in for the year, Agatha and I need to leave for a retreat and vacation in Haaii. For two weeks we'll be staying at a convent retreat house in Maui with some of the sisters from Agatha's community. We'll celebrate Thanksgiving with them. Then for two weeks we'll be in Honolulu at a rented house where we'll join Jim Sanchez's parents. I'm looking forward to getting away and sharing a special time with Agatha. This year has been exhausting and full of challenges to think and pray about from a distance.

I'm not worried about being away for a month. Everything will be in good hands with Emilee. Eric and I are doing better getting along, and our communication has improved. His service and ordeal with the Guard in Afghanistan matured him into a remarkable and responsible son. Considering what he has been through and continues to suffer, I'm grateful he is so willing and able to take charge around here the way he does.

Each year after Mass on All Souls' Day, November 2nd, Eric and I go to the cemetery to place a wreath on his father's grave. When Eric was fifteen, I told him it was his turn to make the wreath for his dad. He devoted a great deal of energy and time to the project which he kept hidden in the shop. On All Souls' morning he put a large cardboard box in the car. I had no idea what to expect until he finally opened the box at the grave. His was no ordinary wreath. It was a plain ring of sharp thorns with no decoration. I didn't say a word. I was beyond a loss for words. We just stood there—those minutes might have been an hour.

This year he told me he was again making the wreath. It went with us in that same cardboard box to Mass and the cemetery. But this time the box contained a wreath of beautiful greens from our property, decorated with cones and a yellow ribbon. He told me he's beginning to think more about his father. Life is different. So is he. So is his father.

Eric and I concluded our visit to the grave with the prayer we have said for many years: "He is safe in God's keeping; so are we."

CHAPTER 32

ERIC

My therapist impressed on me that my unexpected body reactions and sudden anxious thoughts come from my memory scars—from combat and growing up. Aunt Agatha suggested that all this is about the cross I carry...and always will carry. This cross—it's a part of me. I wish this weren't true, that I could somehow leap away from my brain and ditch my wounded self. But as Agatha reminded me, everyone has crosses to carry through life—I'm no exception. She went on to say we're not judged by God because we have crosses; rather, by how well we manage them with God's help and with the help of others in our lives. This is what I was thinking about when I went to bed last night. I said a prayer for Mom and Aunt Agatha over in Hawaii, and for all of us here as I drifted off to sleep.

A vivid dream—not a nightmare—startled me in the middle of the night. I was walking—no shoes and naked—in a dark underground tunnel, holding an oil lantern that gave only a faint glimmer. I have lost my way, my memories. There are faces; I can't make them out. I keep repeating, "Watch your step. Careful. Careful. Where am I going? How much oil is there? Father," I call out, "can't you do this for me? Lord, I surrender. Fill my lantern with oil. There's no cure for a once-torn self other than you." A deep dream voice alerts me. "I provide oil. Keep moving. I am here." With that, I wake up, sit up in bed. Where am I? Who was that?

On the foot of my bed, Prince was curled up and sound asleep. This is the first night since I've been home that he's slept on my bed. He's getting used to me, no longer afraid. We're making progress.

But back to my dream. Think, Eric, I tell myself, what does my dream mean?

I journey in the dark—all alone with nothing but a light—I need that light. Jim's idea about a Higher Power from his AA meetings makes a lot of sense. I need my Higher Power to light my way. I think my dream tells me that without God, I can get lost in the dark. But, those words "I provide oil. Keep moving. I am here" are the words I need to remember and keep.

Throughout my life I have not had a father I could depend on. But now a father has found me—and I have found a father I can trust—my heavenly Father. He will help me live on, give me light to see, strength to care for others, and hopefully lift some weight off my cross.

CHAPTER 33

ERIC

The chilly Thanksgiving morning welcomes the rising sun over Oregon's Willamette Valley. Much of the year's work is now completed and country families are preparing for their traditional reunions with relatives and friends from the city. I asked Emilee, Jim and Jason to get together with me early this morning. I simply told them I have good news and all of them should be in on it.

Jim arrived in the middle of the night after his shift at The Mustang and slept on the couch. Emilee was here at the crack of dawn getting breakfast for everyone. Prince nudged Jason out of bed, and I came in from an early morning walk in the vineyard. We gathered around the kitchen table.

After a few unseemly comments about the condition of the house since Roberta's been away, Emilee asked me what was on my mind. Okay, I said, I've been doing a lot of thinking for a long time about our place here in wine country, and I have some ideas for our future. Before Mom and Aunt Agatha left for Hawaii, we had some good conversations about where we go from here. I think the additional vineyard that Emilee developed this year triggered my thoughts on this. We should now have enough produce to establish our own Stevens Winery. Nobody spoke a word—all wondering what this was leading to.

I continued, I've been so uncertain about my future since I got back from Afghanistan. But I know I'd like to work on a team with the three of you and Mom. For me, working with a great team is the best part of any job or career. Just look at us. It looks like we've got the know-how, the grapes and talent to put out a top brand of Oregon's best wines. Here's the surprise. Our neighbor lady is ready to retire. She's talked to Mom about having us work her property. It could be a great partnership with all the buildings and equipment we'd need. Mom needs all of us to make this work. But, I'm more excited about working with you than anything else. I'm hoping we can all stay together and be close friends. You know, that's what Mom's hoping, too.

While the conversation continued, I couldn't help thinking how the three of us guys each have huge issues that can be frightening. And I bet there will be more tough stuff coming, God help us! But we are honest with one another. Jim's really working on his recovery.

Jason's life is a shambles with all those losses and his divorce. And I'm still struggling with my ghosts. I don't think I could make it without them. Emilee is a rock. She's there for us. We've got to make this work.

Everyone began asking questions at the same time. An atmosphere of excitement filled the kitchen. We can take a chance.

Jason and I went for a walk. Emilee and Jim started getting Thanksgiving dinner ready. Early in the morning, before everyone got up, I set the dining room table with five extra places. They kept asking me about this. In response, I just smiled. It was not long before they had their answer. Major Rodriguez, his wife and three teenagers arrived with a few side dishes to add to our celebration. He already knew I was going to throw out my ideas and assured me of his encouragement and support. Thanksgiving was memorably warm and filled with hope.

P.S. *Jim and I are grateful to the editors of this book for cleaning up our language.*

Love, Eric

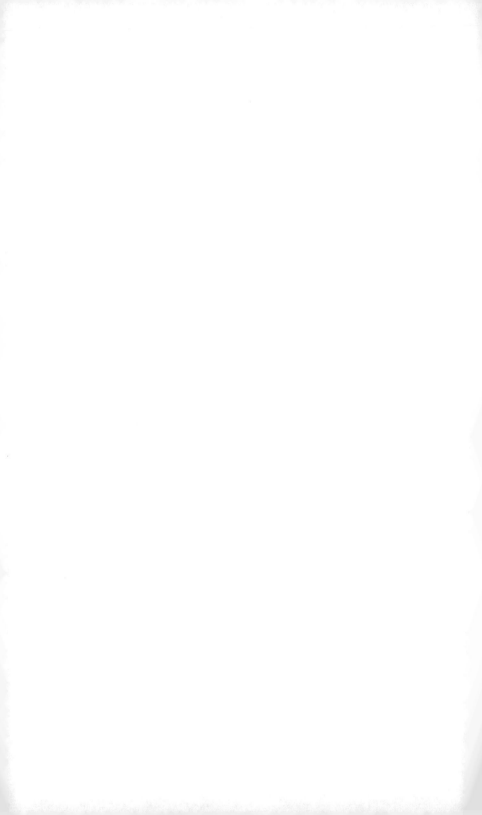

═ Epilogue ═

Our military men and women inspired the creation of this book. It is about scars from PTSD (Post Traumatic Stress Disorder) and mTBI (Mild Traumatic Brain Injury or concussions from explosions) that many suffer as a result of their service in combat. During their stay in a hospital in Portland, Oregon, that treats PTSD, nine active military men were interviewed for this book. Each man contributed confidential information that became a part of the story you read—a story about combat in Afghanistan and coming home—based on actual events in the lives of these men. In some instances, a history of abuse while growing up magnified their scars from combat. Wounds may heal; scars last a lifetime.

At the beginning of our interviews, I asked each man for permission to share some of his personal story. All agreed and assured me that they would be available to provide further help with the book. Our goal,

I told them, is to help people at home understand how PTSD affects relationships and spirituality. We agreed that a story format would be a good way to respect their confidentiality and help others understand.

What is PTSD? If you Google it, more than ten million references will appear! I personally like a description by Colonel Charles Hoge, MD, in his excellent book, *Once a Warrior—Always a Warrior*: "What I'm considering is how each person experiences the condition, or what they perceive the condition to be. For warriors, PTSD can be a day-to-day experience of living with memories they want to forget, staying constantly alert to dangers or perceived dangers others don't pay attention to, enduring sleepless nights, and reacting to things at home as if still in the war zone."

The symptoms of PTSD are usually grouped into three categories: (1) *Re-experiencing* symptoms (flashbacks, bad dreams, frightening thoughts); (2) *Avoidance* symptoms (isolating, feeling emotionally numb, feeling strong guilt or depression, losing interest in activities previously enjoyed, difficulty remembering the dangerous event); and (3) *Hyperarousal* symptoms (being easily startled, feeling tense or on edge, having difficulty sleeping, having angry outbursts).

Mild TBI or concussion symptoms often are temporary and may include some of the following: momentary loss of consciousness, confusion, dizziness, blurred vision, ringing in the ears, fatigue, mood changes, problems with memory, and difficulties with concentration, attention or thinking. Some of these and other aspects of PTSD and mTBI are part of this story.

I am very grateful to all who have assisted with the writing of this book, especially to our military men and women who devote their lives to the service of country and the care of others.

~ Richard Berg, CSC

— Afterword —

I was included in a group of people who received periodic reports from Father Richard Berg, CSC, as he researched this book and interviewed military personnel who had returned from fighting in Iraq and Afghanistan. I live at Mary's Woods retirement community in Lake Oswego, Oregon, where Father Dick is our chaplain. Fr. Dick would often speak about the men and women he was interviewing for this writing project. All of us who heard the stories were touched by the sacrifices and terrible unseen wounds these soldiers had endured while fighting in foreign lands. What was called "shell shock" in World War I and "battle fatigue" in World War II was now defined as Post Traumatic Stress Disorder.

I experienced PTSD up close and personal starting in 2005. My brother, Dick, who was ten years older than I, had been drafted to fight in World War II when I was a young boy and he was merely eighteen years old. He first saw combat in the Battle of the Bulge and continued fighting with the 69th Division until the end of the war. He had been given the Bronze Star and was wounded but refused a Purple Heart at the aid station since he knew it would frighten my mother. After the war, he returned to complete his education and began a life-long career with the Department of the Interior. He and his wife settled in Denver and seemed to live an idyllic and productive middle-class life filled with happiness. Old age brought him deteriorating physical and mental health. After the death of his wife, he was living in a retirement community. The managers reported to me that Dick was losing touch with reality and was hallucinating frequently. Housekeepers would often find five or six wine glasses lined up on his counter. When asked about this, Dick would report they were "for my boys," members of his infantry squad over sixty years ago. My frequent phone calls to him were both sad and frightening. He would often tell me that the President of the United States had sent him and his squad into harm's way to rescue some of our soldiers held by the enemy. I could tell that these incidents were absolutely real to him. Alzheimer's? Hardening of the cerebral arteries? Perhaps—but I believe it was PTSD. The secrets of the war he fought were taken with him to his grave.

The characters in this book represent a broad synthesis of many people Fr. Berg interviewed and spoke with in penetrating detail. Don't presume, however, that the stories told here represent only small, isolated instances of a handful of veterans who are suffering. On the contrary, the Department of Veteran Affairs reports in July 2012 that it is processing a backlog of over 880,000 claims for service, support and compensation. It can be assumed that many of these claims relate in some way to PTSD. We often wring our hands over the deaths suffered in the wars fought in Iraq and Afghanistan. While these losses are truly terrible, the number of brave men and women who have died is but a fraction of all those who have suffered possible lifelong injuries—many of which are not related to physical wounds. No, the characters in this book represent a microscopic view of an enormous problem. It is our job to raise awareness about this most serious situation.

But, what can I—a solitary individual—do to make a difference? As Fr. Berg is quick to tell those in his congregation, we can all pray for those afflicted with this syndrome. The scriptural call to love our neighbor includes earnestly entreating God on their behalf. Each of us can also devote some time to raising awareness and being of actual help to our veterans. A simple Internet search will reveal many local organizations, both private and public, that are offering assistance to vets suffering PTSD. Finally, some can also share their treasure. There are many worthwhile, well-managed organizations that can effectively use your contributions to assist these medically struggling veterans. May all of us, vets and non-vets alike, develop a better personal awareness of the terrible injuries faced by those who have stepped forward to defend the national interests of the United States of America. God bless them all!

~ Greg Hadley